Surrender... or Fight?

One Woman's Victory over Cancer

Beatrice Hofman Hoek
and
Melanie Jongsma

Baker Books

A Division of Baker Book House Co
Grand Rapids, Michigan 49516

Library of Congress Cataloging-in-Publication Data

Hoek, Beatrice Hofman, 1941–
    Surrender . . . or Fight? : one woman's victory over cancer /
Beatrice Hofman Hoek and Melanie Jongsma.
        p. cm.
    ISBN 0-8010-4401-4
    1. Hoek, Beatrice, 1941– . 2. Breast—Cancer—Patients—
Biography. 3. Breast—Cancer—Patients—Religious life. 4. Cancer—
Religious aspects—Christianity. I. Jongsma, Melanie, 1967–   .
II. Title.
    RC280.B8H625   1995
    362.1'9699'4490092—dc20
    [B]   94-31021

Unless otherwise indicated, Scripture quotations are from the HOLY BIBLE, NEW INTERNATIONAL VERSION ® NIV ®.Copyright 1973, 1978, 1984 by International Bible Society. Used by permission of Zondervan Publishing House. All rights reserved. Other versions used are KIng James Version (KJV) and The Living Bible (LB).

Contents

Contents

Foreword

Those of us who know Bea Hoek are pleased that she has taken the time to share her cancer experience with a broader circle. This brief and touching book will enable many to benefit from the way she has handled the terror and depression that accompany the cancer battle.

Each of the diseases we are prey to has its characteristic impact on its victims. Heart patients are often quite tense and even rebellious because their disease requires that they change their lifestyle. Cancer patients, in contrast, seem to develop a resignation, even a sweetness about themselves. The disease of cancer requires those who have it to think totally differently about their bodies than they did before. It's not just that one organ is diseased, but cancer serves notice that the entire organism is fundamentally flawed. Cancer announces that these precious bodies of ours cannot cope with whatever it is that is caus-ing cell growth to run amok. It is very, very humiliating. Even embarrassing.

Bea Hoek talks about this. And she talks about the loneliness. It is a peculiar kind of loneliness, experienced, in her case, while her husband and children and church family loved and cared for her. It is the loneliness that comes from realizing that you must carry on the battle all by yourself.

In this book we learn that the cancer experience has its good side. For Bea Hoek it brought her to the point of total surrender, a surrender that enables her now to deal with her enemy's reappearance. Currently, her battle is going well, and she has reason to hope for the future. But it is very unsettling to live with this uncertainty.

And cancer patients realize that the uncertainty that never leaves them is really the way it is for everyone. There is no place of certain refuge this side of glory. Bea learned that one fateful day in October 1983, and she has learned her lesson well.

A cancer patient finally comes to the place where his of her hope is in God and God alone. And, of course, that is where it should be for all of us—all the time.

For believers the good side of cancer is that it brings them to that strange and wonderful place where they discover that God perfects his strength in their weakness. They learn to be thankful and happy even when November days are repeatedly without sunshine.

Foreword

Those of us who know Bea Hoek are grateful for the testimony that follows and join together in prayer that God will continue to give her the splendor of his victory. We know he will.

Joel Nederhood
Director of Ministries
The Back to God Hour/Faith 20

Introduction

$\mathcal{I}$ *am Bea's doctor.* I just finished reading her book, and I am proud to be part of Bea's life. I am proud because Bea has taught me much about how a Christian (a deeply committed, vibrant, and emotional Christian) fights cancer. I am proud because Bea is alive and possibly free of cancer. I am proud because the treatments have allowed her to maintain her body image, in spite of the scars. I am proud because she has grown in faith and strength, and she has been an example to those around her (especially to those of us who knew her when we were both younger).

In other ways, though, I feel embarrassed and awkward. I am embarrassed because Bea has reminded me that I am not always the best doctor I can be; sometimes I am cross, arrogant, or too busy. Sometimes I am skeptical when I should be supportive. And some-

Introduction

times I am just plain wrong. For example, I look back at the use of prednisone for Bea's breast cancer in 1983, and I realize now that the medicine probably wasn't necessary. It certainly contributed significantly to her emotional swings and some of the other side effects.

I am also embarrassed because I wasn't more optimistic when we started. Breast cancer patients with ten or more lymph nodes affected, as Bea had, are generally given a guarded prognosis, and I chose to be "realistic" rather than hopeful.

I am embarrassed because I was skeptical of Bea's "special diets." We in the medical profession are now beginning to realize that low fat, high fiber diets are important in cancer prevention and may slow the growth of some cancers.

I am embarrassed because I did not take seriously Bea's emotional ups and downs. I laughed them off at times when I should have recognized them as very real symptoms of a physical, spiritual, and emotional struggle.

Most of all, I am embarrassed because through this all Bea was and is a more vibrant Christian than I am. Bea lets her light shine! As a professional in a big urban hospital, though, I cloak myself in sedate restraint and only occasionally let my faith speak out.

So in conclusion, Bea has taught me much. She has taught me that the love of our heavenly Father extends into every part of our lives—not just in church, home, and school, but also in work, in the chemotherapy suite, under the radiation machine, or in the operating room. He is here with us all the time and will help us through any uncertainty, through any waiting, if we will simply and totally surrender ourselves to his love. Please read this book. It's short and it's sweet.

Nicholas J. Vogelzang, M.D.
Professor of Medicine
University of Chicago Hospitals

I Surrender All

All to Jesus I surrender,
all to him I freely give;
I will ever love and trust him,
in his presence daily live.

All to Jesus I surrender.
Make me, Savior, wholly thine.
Let me feel the Holy Spirit—
truly know that thou art mine.

All to Jesus I surrender.
Lord, I give myself to thee.
Fill me with thy love and power,
let thy blessings fall on me.

I surrender all.
I surrender all.
All to thee, my blessed Savior,
I surrender all.

–Judson W. Van de Venter

1
A Glimpse of How It All Turns Out

October 1992. I sat next to my husband in church last Sunday. On the other side of me was my granddaughter, and filling the rest of the pew were my parents, my youngest daughter, and my son and daughter-in-law.

It was a communion Sunday, a day of celebration. The elements were passed, and I watched each member of my family, one by one, accept the body and blood of Christ. When my own turn came, my eyes filled with tears. God's goodness was almost too much for me to bear.

Nine years ago I had been diagnosed with cancer. After nonchalantly signing into a local clinic to have a lump checked out, I was virtually unprepared for the reality of cancer. In fact, I responded to the doctor's pronouncement by fainting.

Within the next few days I entered the hospital for a biopsy. When I awoke from the anesthesia, two of my three children were standing at my bedside with a few close friends. I was told the tumor was malignant, and I remember telling the kids that this was "God's will," but actually my faith had been devastated. Throughout that night—and many nights to follow—I woke up and prayed, "Lord, please don't let me die." I was only forty-two. I wanted to see my children graduate from high school. I wanted to celebrate my twenty-fifth wedding anniversary with the man I loved. I wanted grandchildren and retirement—all the normal things.

Looking back now I realize that I had never really known or understood the grace of God. I had been a committed Christian, perhaps even a woman of faith, but that faith was tender and untested. The next few years would add depth and meaning to my faith through trials that would have paralyzed me with fear had I known about them in advance.

A lumpectomy, nine months of chemotherapy, twenty-eight days of radiation with second-degree burns, lymph node surgery, radiation implant surgery, and always the interminable waiting—this is what my immediate future held. Then, after years of remission, the cancer came back. Several months of oral chemotherapy, as well as another round of intense soul-searching, followed. Through it all, the only thing I had to hold on to was God's promise to keep me "in perfect peace whose mind is stayed on thee" (Isa. 26:3 KJV).

The past nine years have been a struggle not only against cancer but also against all the exhausting emotions that go along with it. I have suffered pain, sickness, dependence, fear, and humiliation. I have plumbed the depths of my faith in God with every ounce of strength and courage I have.

But God's grace has been sufficient for me. And I came to understand that only by totally surrendering myself to it.

Last Sunday I sat in church with my family, and I cried with joy. Perhaps confused by my tears, my little granddaughter looked up at me and smiled. All I could do was breathe a prayer of thanks and hug her.

2
A Normal Life

October 1983. I was well into school, church, and family activities—loving it all, yet feeling overwhelmed at times. I was taking a class at a nearby university. I was doing telephone counseling for a church-related television outreach program called *Faith 20* one morning a month. I was volunteering in the Career Opportunities Program at the high school. I was teaching Sunday school. All this besides the normal busy-ness of raising two high-schoolers and a sixth-grader, and being involved in *their* activities. Perhaps I had taken on too much.

Jon, my oldest son, was a high school senior. He was into fixing cars and trucks—taking them apart and putting them back together, over and over again. He spent countless hours in the garage with his friends, while I spent time in the kitchen putting together cookies and milk to offer them.

Jayne was a sophomore in high school, and she was immersed in friends, sports, and other activities. I seem to remember spending a lot of time in the lobby of the orthodontist's office that year, too. Our house was always full of Jayne's group of girlfriends. And our evenings and weekends were often spent driving them around.

Jackie was a sixth-grade sports fanatic. She tried out for every team she could think of, and made most of them. When she wasn't at a tryout or a practice or a game of some sort, she was at a friend's birthday party or a sleepover. She was also learning to balance her active social life with the responsibility of a paper route.

My husband, Jim, was an instrumental music director for a nearby school district. His involvement with church committees, a local choir, and two part-time jobs added to the frantic pace our whole family seemed to be caught up in that year.

I remember specifically Saturday, October 15. My tight weekend schedule would not provide any reprieve from the week's activities, and I was simply overwhelmed. My prayer that day was, "Lord, slow me down. This pace is too hectic for me."

I don't know if the events that followed were God's way of answering that prayer. But less than two weeks later, my life changed, and I haven't been the same since.

3
The Shock of Diagnosis

*O*nly *nine days* after that prayer I found a lump in my left breast. It was a rather large lump, and I found it accidentally. Being only forty-two years old—what I felt was the prime of life—I had never paid much attention to doctors' scoldings about checking yourself regularly. I was feeling fine. I was going strong. But God had other plans for me.

I didn't waste any time making an appointment for an examination. Though I was worried, I was not overly alarmed. After all, I had heard about the benefits of early detection.

Two days later was Grandparents Day at the high school, and my parents had come from Wisconsin for the occasion. I casually told them of my discovery as I dropped them off at the school. I then nonchalantly signed into the local clinic, taking along my Sunday school lesson so I could study while waiting. The time passed quickly, and after about twenty minutes my name was called.

It was only then that my attention turned to the issue at hand. The room was small and stuffy, and the doctor—smelling of cigarette smoke—was rather brusque. He was probably a good surgeon, though he seemed to have a difficult time relating to people's emotions, communicating his sympathy, or both.

I explained that I had found the lump in my left breast and asked if I should be concerned about it. He responded with a few questions of his own, examined the lump, and decided to try to aspirate it (draw fluid from it). I winced at the size of the needle and wondered how this was going to work. He inserted the needle slowly and attempted to draw out any fluid, but there was no fluid to draw. Without his telling me, I knew what that meant. This was a possible malignancy. I fainted.

A few minutes later the doctor had revived me with smelling salts. When I had regained some composure he began talking about cancer—using words like *biopsy, mastectomy, chemotherapy,* and *radiation.* My mind was spinning, and I could not even grasp the information I was hearing. *"There has to be a better way to give someone this news,"* I thought.

(Today doctors are mandated by law in several states to carefully discuss treatment options with their patients. In Michigan, for example, the "Breast Cancer Informed Consent Law" requires doctors to provide a brochure to each patient they diagnose as having breast cancer. The brochure offers simple yet detailed information about the disease and its different treatment approaches, as well as definitions of various medical terms.)

I remember telling the doctor that I wanted to research my options and that I wanted a second opinion as soon as possible. But without being overt, he tried to pressure me to choose a mastectomy. Of course, he was a surgeon, and naturally, he felt most comfortable with a surgical remedy, so no other options were discussed.

I walked out of the small room almost in a nightmare. *"This can't be a serious problem,"* I argued with myself. *"I'm not sick, and I'm young. I can't have cancer."* But as reality slowly filtered through my denial, I began to feel very vulnerable and alone.

I wandered over to the cashier to settle my account, hardly even aware of what I was doing. My world had changed, and I hadn't adjusted yet. I walked out of the clinic and into the parking lot in a daze.

Two days later I visited another surgeon in the same clinic. He was kind and very sympathetic, much more

so than the doctor who had given me the news. Still,
this second doctor gave me the same opinion—a
biopsy at a local hospital and then a mastectomy if
the tumor was malignant. I left quickly and broke into
tears once inside my car. In fear, uncertainty, and anxiety I cried out, *"Lord, I don't know what you are doing
in my life right now, but please don't leave me. Help
me trust you."*

How Firm a Foundation

How firm a foundation, you saints of the Lord,
  is laid for your faith in his excellent word!
What more can he say than to you he has said,
  to you who for refuge to Jesus have fled?

"Fear not, I am with you; O be not dismayed,
  for I am your God and will still give you aid;
I'll strengthen you, help you, and cause you to stand,
  upheld by my righteous, omnipotent hand.

"The soul that on Jesus has leaned for repose
  I will not, I will not desert to its foes.
That soul, though all hell should endeavor to shake,
  I'll never, no never, no never forsake!"

—J. Rippon

4
Responding

There are three possible responses to a cancer diagnosis. You can go home, draw the shades, curl up under a blanket, and prepare to die. Even without being that obvious or morbid about it, you make it clear to yourself and others that you have decided not to fight. Sure, you accept your treatment program and continue your doctor visits, but the absence of an inner drive to become healthy again, and the confidence that recovery is possible, turn your treatments into little more than hollow ritual.

Another response is to be positive, strong, and continually optimistic, prepared to fight and confident of victory. You overcome your fear by denying the possibility of death. *"I can overcome it—there's nothing*

24

to be afraid of," you tell yourself. *"It's mind over matter, and if I don't let it get to me, it won't."*

But the third response lies somewhere in the middle. You acknowledge reality, admit that you might in fact die, and then go ahead and fight anyway. It is only natural to feel afraid and powerless in the face of terminal illness, and there is nothing wrong with expressing those feelings. But at the same time, no good comes of giving up.

Even so, deciding to fight does not guarantee that you will never again feel like giving up. Much of the battle vacillates between feelings of helplessness and confidence. It is difficult to find the middle ground.

After hearing my diagnosis, I was totally overwhelmed. I said to myself, *"It would be easier to die than to face multiple surgeries, chemotherapy, radiation, needles, and then uncertainty."* I understood why some cancer victims give up. I could even imagine why some cancer patients commit suicide. The grief and fear are almost inexpressible. The pain doesn't go away. The despair and anxiety are all-consuming. There is no way out on one's own.

But my second reaction was to hang on tightly to my God, whom I had always claimed as the Lord of my life. He is the only ray of hope in a situation that feels hopeless. He is the only source of life—even in the face of death.

The battle would be fierce between the enemy and me. But with God's help I began to fight with every ounce of strength and courage I had.

5
The Journey Begins

After receiving two professional opinions in favor of a mastectomy, I was discouraged but not hopeless. My former pastor, Rev. Vogelzang, had a son, Nick, a well-known doctor, and I turned to him for alternatives. Over the phone he told me he had some new information and would get back to me in an hour or so. I had no idea what this "new information" was, but somehow I was encouraged. I eagerly anticipated his return call that evening.

The call came, and Dr. Vogelzang gave me my options: If the tumor was malignant, I could choose to have either a mastectomy (removal of the breast) or a lumpectomy (removal of the lump and surrounding tissue, also called breast preservation). If I chose a mastectomy, a silicone breast implant was possible some months after surgery. Chemotherapy would be necessary if the lymph nodes were involved. If I chose a lumpectomy, I would still need nine months of chemo, as well as five and a half weeks of external radiation, and internal radiation implant surgery would also be possible.

Although today this kind of information is given routinely, for me it was the first professional confirmation I'd had that my situation wasn't totally dark. Hearing a number of alternatives from a doctor I knew I could trust lifted my spirits. It seemed I had forgotten what hope felt like, and now it came rushing back. God was still right there with me.

One thing I have learned and relearned throughout my experience is the beauty and importance of the body of Christ. When one becomes a Christian and joins God's family, he or she has access to God's power and friendship—not only in a vertical "me-to-God" sense, but also in a horizontal "me-to-God's-people" sense. I checked into the hospital that Sunday in preparation for my biopsy, and when I entered my room, I found God's presence in a Christian woman and her visiting husband, who offered to pray with me.

My husband and I, and Ramona Moore (my room-mate) and her husband lifted our hearts to God together. We poured out our fears and prayed for healing. We asked for faith and repeated the promises we had all been raised on. We felt God's Spirit within us and among us, and we were strengthened by it.

Monday morning dawned, the day of my biopsy. The prayer support I had received from the Moores and others, as well as the time I had spent reading some of the psalms, left me feeling peacefully prepared for my upcoming surgery. A nurse started the intravenous, and I was wheeled off to the operating room.

6
That Doesn't Mean It's Easy

The biopsy (one of the meanest) completed, I was full of morphine. What is today often a twenty-minute out-patient procedure, was back then major surgery. The resulting physical pain, nausea, and weariness had robbed me of the peace I had felt a few hours before. All I wanted was sleep. I dozed fitfully until my husband Jim and my two high school-aged children came in with four of their friends. My husband had met them in the parking lot and had given them the latest news. Now they stood with me while I was filled in. The tumor was malignant.

My journal entry for that day says, "My world crashed, but God is in control." I groggily mouthed to the kids something about God's will, but my spirit was devastated. I sat up, and the room seemed to ripple and spin. Maybe my dizziness and nausea were the only things that kept me from total despair. I was so tired and sick that I could not get a good mental or emotional grasp on what was happening to me.

I checked out of the hospital on Tuesday and immediately secured an appointment for Thursday with Dr. Vogelzang at the University of Chicago Hospital. I had already decided to have the lymph node surgery and radiation implant surgery (which involved a seventy-two-hour isolation period) at a hospital in Decatur. Radiation implant surgery or internal radiation (the insertion of iridium-filled rods) is no longer necessary today because external radiation is much more effective. But back then, radiation implants were almost necessary to insure that all of the cancer was targeted. I discussed my plan with Dr. Vogelzang, who had first provided me with information about the Decatur hospital. The following day, Friday, Jim and I made our first trip to Decatur.

Decatur Memorial Hospital had a peaceful and professional atmosphere about it. As soon as I walked in the front doors, I felt confident about the care I would receive. We met with both the lymph node surgeon and the implant surgeon, a man who had studied in

30

Paris for two years. The entire consultation was very reassuring, and we left Decatur with high hopes.

On the way home we stopped at a restaurant with my parents. It was their wedding anniversary, and they wanted to treat us to dinner. I was happy for them, but I couldn't help feeling sorry for myself at the same time. The peace and confidence I had felt during my surgery consultation dissipated. The longing for a normal life returned, along with the fear that I might not be able to celebrate another year with my husband. A cold chill settled over me, and I tried to enjoy the dinner, but I couldn't concentrate. My life seemed joyless.

Meaningful relationships have less to do with emotion than with commitment. This is true in our human relationships as well as our relationship with God. There were few times during my battle with cancer that I *felt* powerful, but I knew the power was there for me to tap into. There were many times when I felt angry or scared or anxious or hopeless, but I remained committed to God and the belief that he could heal me. I have learned that joy is not an emotion; it is something deeper. Often I have prayed, "In spite of how I feel, Lord, I will find my hope and joy in you." And I *know* he has never left me, even though there were times when I *felt* he had.

When we arrived home that evening, we proceeded to make arrangements for surgery and testing in Decatur. Since we wanted to begin as soon as possible, there wasn't much time, but the family of God surrounded us again, and we quickly found friends for the kids to stay with.

We left the next morning, Sunday, and arrived that afternoon. It was important to find out if the cancer was primarily in my breast, or if it had spread, so a liver and spleen scan was scheduled for Monday. In the meantime, the doctor came to my room and spent a few minutes asking questions, giving answers, and generally reassuring us. By the time he left, we were feeling peaceful and confident again. Jim and I then united our hearts in a private prayer together.

Jim was able to stay in a guest room at the hospital for the entire week. His closeness had a stabilizing effect on my emotional health, and I thank the Lord that he generously provided everything he knew I would need.

The liver and spleen scan on Monday went well, and the tests came back clear. On Tuesday I went through a bone scan and a CAT scan. I was supposed to receive an injection of radioactive dye, but for some reason my veins would not accept it. The needle punctured my skin tissue, and the dye began to burn under my skin. The pain was severe. Knowing this was not a normal reaction did not make it any easier to deal with. I wanted to forget the whole thing, but I couldn't. Crying to relieve the tension, I prayed and recited a verse from the psalms: "What time I am afraid, I will put my trust in you." Finally the dye was inserted and the test could proceed.

Because the LORD is my Shepherd, I have everything I need!

He lets me rest in the meadow grass and leads me beside the quiet streams. He gives me new strength. He helps me do what honors him the most.

Even when walking through the dark valley of death I will not be afraid, for you are close beside me, guarding, guiding all the way.

You provide delicious food for me in the presence of my enemies. You have welcomed me as your guest; blessings overflow!

Your goodness and unfailing kindness shall be with me all of my life, and afterwards I will live with you forever in your home.

—Psalm 23 LB

To me the CAT scan machine was huge and intimidating. I entered head-first, lying helpless on the table and feeling completely alone. But even in the heart of that cold, computerized instrument, God reminded me, "Lo, I am with you always, even to the end of the world." We may place our faith in science and technology, but God's power goes beyond human technology. Again, the tests came back clear. Again, I thanked my God.

Lymph node surgery was scheduled for the next day. The outcome of this surgery was a key factor in my diagnosis. The entire procedure was completed in an hour and a half, and seventeen lymph nodes were removed. Ten of them tested positive.

Not only were the lymph nodes infected but the cancer cells had invaded my bloodstream as well. My doctor said he was very concerned, and I figured that was good reason for me to be concerned. Our attack would have to be aggressive. My treatment would include chemotherapy every two weeks for nine months, twenty-eight days of external radiation, and finally radiation implant surgery.

My emotional strength had faltered at the news of the test results, but my commitment to and dependence on God drew me to his feet in prayer. I begged for continued mercy.

7
Not a Lonely Battle

Dealing with people after the news gets out about your serious diagnosis can be both frustrating and exhilarating. It is difficult enough to sort through your own emotions, but I often felt as though I also had to deal with the emotions of everyone around me.

Reactions are widely varied. Some people feel so much pain for you that they can hardly approach you, let alone engage in conversation. They view you from a distance, very cautiously, trying to calculate how you might be handling this trial. I have found that when *I* approach *them* with a "Hi! How are you?" the nervous discomfort is more quickly relieved. I guess people just need you to convince them that you are your normal self, especially when you're not.

Some people ask questions, others give hugs, some have tears in their eyes, and many mention that they are praying for you. Everyone handles the illness of a friend in a different way, and all are important reinforcements for you as you enter the thick of the battle.

Somehow when you make the decision to fight, people are encouraged. Once you become a cancer patient you become a reminder of mortality, a reality most people try to deny. But your fighting back seems to make it easier for them to deal with their own feelings.

In a sense, all of us are alone. Because each of us is unique—in personality, in background, in the trials we face—none of us can ever truly understand what someone else is thinking and feeling and experiencing. Whether it's cancer or dealing with an alcoholic father or raising a retarded child or overcoming feelings of inadequacy, each of us faces a unique life situation. Each of us is alone. In that sense, I was alone with my cancer. No one else in the world could understand what I was going through.

> Turn to me and be gracious to me,
> for I am lonely and afflicted.
> The troubles of my heart have multiplied;

free me from my anguish.
Look upon my affliction
and my distress
and take away all my sins.
—Psalm 25:16-18

But in another sense, we Christians are never alone, because we are part of the body of Christ. Although our functions and situations are unique, we are all intricately bound together by his love and his ultimate purpose.

The love I felt from the family of God was a source of strength throughout my struggle. Some people brought me food, flowers, or books; others gave clothing, pictures, or cassette tapes. Some helped with household chores or made themselves available to answer the phone. A beautician friend donated a perm to my younger daughter. Another friend gave my older daughter spending money for a school outing when I was hospitalized. Yet another was able to take my daughter to piano lessons each week. And many people offered financial assistance.

Cards, notes, and phone calls from all over the country reminded me of the constant prayers people were offering in my behalf. A faraway friend wrote that people I didn't even know were praying for me. One of the kindest things said to me was, "I don't know exactly what you're going through, but I feel your pain." I was not alone.

If you know someone who is being treated for cancer, let the person know he or she is not alone.

Don't be afraid to reach out with the talents and resources you have to offer—including emotional resources like hugs and smiles. If you find it hard to deal with your friend's illness, at least send a card on a regular basis. Pray faithfully, and let your friend *know* you are praying.

On the other hand, if you are battling cancer yourself, don't be ashamed to invite other people into the fight with you. Don't be embarrassed about your own limitations. Don't be too proud to accept the help others offer. Not only does admitting your weaknesses free you from feeling that you have to hide them, it also provides your friends an escape from the helplessness many of them will feel. It is difficult to suffer alone, but it may be just as difficult to watch someone else suffer without being able to help.

Even if you find that you cannot allow yourself to depend on the people around you—for whatever reason—you can take comfort in knowing that you still do not have to face cancer alone. God promises to join you in the struggle whenever you ask him.

It was not a lonely battle for me. It doesn't have to be for anyone.

8
Kind Words
from a Friend

*J*oel Nederhood is a well-known pastor in our area, and he has been a friend for a long time. During my ordeal, Joel provided our family with a great deal of emotional support and spiritual advice—through letters, phone calls, and personal visits. The rest of this chapter is taken from a letter he sent me in November 1983. I have kept it for all these years because it still means so much to me. I found his words so helpful that I have read and reread this letter over and over again:

Surrender . . . or Fight?

Dear Bea,

I thought I would put down some of my thoughts about your case on paper, because this will give you an opportunity to think about some of these things occasionally over the next weeks and months. I've done a lot of thinking about cancer, as you know, and since I had my operation and therapy, so many people who have had cancer have come up to me and have opened their hearts to me.

. . . First of all, I would just like to urge you to keep up your courage and to battle your cancer with all of the resources at your disposal. I realize that you have been disappointed because some of the lymph nodes were infected and you know, of course, that you have a form of cancer that will have to be attacked aggressively. . . . What you are involved in is a battle, pure and simple. The enemy must be understood and its location pinpointed; and the weapons must be designed to destroy this enemy. And with all this, so much depends on your own determination to get on with the battle.

There is much to hope for. I am always impressed with the survivors I meet. I talk with people who were nearly destroyed by cancer ten years ago, and they are doing well today. A young man, about thirty-five years old, sat in my office just the other day, and we rejoiced together because of the way God had healed him. He had discovered his lymphoma himself, and the tumors were so numerous there was no thought of operating. He had chemotherapy at Mayo's and has been free from cancer now for more than three years.

I want to emphasize that surviving is a real possibility, no matter how virulent one's cancer is. And we as Christians feel this especially because we know that our great God does not surrender to the forces of evil no matter how formidable these forces may be. You are a woman of faith, and we may know right now that whatever happens, he will glorify himself in your sickness. Right now we have every reason to pray and work for healing. So far as we can see, from our human perspective, you have work to do for the Savior yet within this world. Claim Psalm 118:17–18 as your very own: "I will not die but live, and will proclaim what the LORD has done. The LORD has chastened me severely, but he has not given me over to death."

. . . When we talked on the phone the other day, you asked whether I thought you should get out and do some of the errands that you had to do. I strongly feel that you should do just as much as you can, even when you are having your chemotherapy. I suppose you will be sick for a day or so every time you have your chemo. But once that wears off, do your work, be a housewife and a mother to your children. Obviously, if you are too ill to do such things, you automatically will not do them. But if you have some strength, use it. There was an article in the *Reader's Digest* two years ago or perhaps even longer, which told of a man who was having chemotherapy, and he continued with his running. I don't suppose he ran as much or as long as before, but he didn't sit around and act like a sick person. Try to maintain your normal schedule. Go to church, go to societies, life must go on, and we are all praying that what you are going through now will be only a detour, and by this time next year you will be back at your regular activities.

With all of this, I would encourage you to be as positive as you can be about this experience in its totality. There is so much to it. There is the trauma that accompanies the diagnosis, there is the weakness and mutilation associated with the surgery, there is the nausea and other side effects of the therapy, there is the long exposure to the world of doctors and medicine and hospitals, there is the relationship with your friends, with your family and with Jim. There is your own psyche, the deep, deep feelings which sometimes will cause you to weep. A person like you is an injured, fearsome, human being who is being forced to face up to facts about your mortality that most of us succeed in putting out of our minds most of the time.

41

Surrender . . . or Fight?

The cancer experience is unique. And you are right in the middle of it at this moment, and you will plunge even deeper into it over the next months. View all this as a learning process. You will learn so much—so much about yourself, so much about others. You will meet people you would never have met before. Possibly you will be able to speak to them about the Savior. In any case, you are going through something while you are still a young person, and if you survive, you will be able to be of enormous help to others. So (I hardly dare say this), savor the experience. This experience has its own excitement and its own reward.

This is not an easy thing—making the most of the experience. . . . What little there is that is pleasant in the cancer experience is bittersweet; and most of it is the very opposite of pleasant. But there is a sense of being close to the essence of life as a person is forced to come face to face with exactly what kind of a person he or she is. All this is, as Philip Yancey has put it, a gift nobody wants. But it is a gift, even so; a gift from God.

Yes, God—where is God in all this? How hard it is to answer this question, but God is with us when we go through these things. When we are weak, he perfects his strength in our bodies, in our lives. Nothing happens outside his *fatherly* control. I emphasize fatherly, for we must never allow ourselves to think about God without remembering that he is our Father. Not a hair shall fall from our heads without his knowledge. (Now, there's something for a cancer patient who sees his or her hair disappear.) God is with us always. And the events of our individual lives are carefully designed for us. Each of us must live his/her own life. Each of us has a different life. But your life, too, is under his direction. This present testing, this, too, is part of the perfect pattern of your earthly experience. It is something your heavenly Father is using to prepare you for that eternal existence in which there will be no sickness and no tears.

Above all else, this is a time in which you can plumb the depths of the Christian faith as you never have before.

And Jim and your children can join you in this. There is a comfort in Christianity that is without limit. There is as much there as we want to use. This is a time to live with Jesus, the great high priest who sacrificed himself through the most painful and shameful death on the cross. This is a time in which prayer becomes so much more than something we happen to do occasionally, but it becomes the most fundamental speech we utter. What do we have if we do not have prayer? But we do have prayer. And we do not know exactly what God's answer to our specific requests will be, but we do know that the Almighty God who has made everything hears—he hears! "The eyes of the LORD are on the righteous and his ears are attentive to their cry. . . . The righteous cry out, and the LORD hears them; he delivers them from all their troubles" (Psalm 34:15, 17).

So you pray, Jim prays, your children learn to pray as never before, your friends do—we pray for your healing—that God will use the means. We pray for your faith that it will remain strong no matter what. And we all rest in the understanding that whatever happens in your life does not happen off in a corner somewhere where his gaze does not penetrate. He sees you, he sees everything that is going on, and he loves you—just now when you feel so helpless, you may know that God loves you.

This is ultimately where we end as we go through the valley as Christians—we know, we know, that nothing can separate us from the love of God that is in Christ Jesus our Lord (Rom. 8:39). This is an absolute statement—nothing can separate us. Nothing. Not even cancer. Not even death. And not even life. Nothing can.

Bea, all of us, your friends, surrender you prayerfully to the love of God and we are sure that you are safe with him.

> Sincerely, in Christ,
> Joel Nederhood

9
Fighting Back

So, once I had decided to fight back, what did I do? What exactly did it mean to "fight back" against an enemy like cancer?

It was easy to feel like I was not in control of my life after cancer entered it. The cancer seemed to take over everything. My time was no longer my own—my schedule now revolved around treatments and appointments. My thoughts weren't my own—the cancer filled my mind despite my efforts to think about anything else. My emotions were controlled by both the cancer and whatever drugs were a part of my treatment. Even my body wasn't my own—after surgery and weight loss and nausea and the disease itself, I didn't look much like the person I used to be.

But there were practical, concrete things I found I could do to fight the cancer. These are the things I think were largely responsible for my recovery.

Prayer

I cannot overemphasize my dependence on God. Not only did I learn to talk to God honestly and meaningfully, I also learned to *listen* to him. I searched the Bible for his messages to me. I listened to inspiring music. I attended church as often as I could. And God did not let me down. When I needed comfort, his message was gentle. When I needed discipline, his reminders were clear. Every time I turned to him, he spoke to me and told me just what I needed to hear.

Writing down your prayers or praying with a partner may help keep you focused during a time when you have a lot on your mind.

You may feel at times that you simply cannot pray—your emotions are drained and your heart is empty. At those times, try using the Bible as your prayer book. Many of the psalms, for example, are expressions of intense dependence on God. You may find that they express your inexpressible feelings.

Acceptance

I could not fight a disease if I refused to admit I had it. I had to face my enemy head-on. This was no time to flinch from reality. At the same time, acknowledging cancer's power did not mean resigning myself to it.

Possible responses were one of these three:

Denial. "This isn't so tough; I can easily beat it."
Resignation. "This is tough; I'll never beat it."
Acceptance. "This is tough; I'll have to work hard to beat it."

Accepting my cancer meant walking the thin line between denial and resignation.

Knowledge

I made myself as well-informed as I could about my disease. I talked to my doctor. I asked questions. I joined groups. I read books. I listened to other cancer patients. Even watching movies about another person's battle was helpful to me.

I made myself a partner with my doctor. I entered into the decision-making process instead of simply "following orders."

Obedience

Still, I did religiously follow the regimen my doctor prescribed for me. This meant not only taking the proper medications at the proper times but also meticulously following his orders regarding diet, exercise, and general well-being.

I found *Fit for Life* (1987) to be a strong argument for a very strict, healthy diet. The book recommends avoiding any food that is packaged in a box, can, or bag, and filling up instead on fruits, vegetables, and whole grains. It's also healthy to drink plenty of liquids: eight glasses of pure water each day, as well as unsweetened fruit juices.

Exercise is important, too. You may feel too weak to lift weights or run marathons, but exercise doesn't have to be exhausting. I often would take a casual stroll around the block, or through the forest preserve. I tried to spend time outdoors. For me it was really not all that important *what* I did, as long as I did *something*, and did it regularly, setting goals for myself and working to meet them. Just getting myself off the couch or out of bed, getting dressed, and stepping out the front door was a positive step. It symbolized my refusal to accept cancer's hold on my life.

Actively involving oneself in becoming whole is essential. Exercise is not only a symbolic step toward health, or only a way to build up muscular strength and aerobic endurance, it has also been proven to stimulate the body's immune system. It takes determination and discipline to achieve a regular schedule of physical activity, but is well worth the effort.

Positive thinking

I surrounded myself with positive people, people who were willing to accept the seriousness of my illness without losing hope, that is, people who were willing to walk the thin line of acceptance with me. I relied on those friends who could help me deal with my cancer without making it the center of every conversation. I spent time with people who would do normal, everyday things with me. I even looked for the humorous side to catastrophe. "Laugh often," I reminded myself. Remember, there is no type of cancer that does not have some rate of recovery.

It was important for me to regain and/or maintain as many of my regular activities as I could. This gave me a sense of normalcy, kept my mind off the cancer, and helped me avoid thinking like a victim. I refused to waste time in bed all morning. I got up and took charge of my day. Also, I tried every day to look my best, because then I felt better, too.

Positive thinking relates to prayer and Bible reading, too. When I found an uplifting, inspirational verse in the Bible, I copied it onto a note card and taped it up where I would see it often. I tried to remember to pray out my thanksgiving and praise as well as my tears and anxieties. I listened to inspirational music. I watched sit-coms on TV. And I read light books and magazines.

Support

I cannot overemphasize the role my husband played in my recovery. As I recuperated from that first surgery in the Decatur hospital, Jim and I shared a special closeness and began forging a bond that would withstand all of the fear and frustration and weariness that we didn't even know were yet to come. We spent many hours alone together, trying to come to grips with our new life and our changing relationship with each other.

I did not let my family and friends abandon me. I asked for help and understanding, but not pity. I was not a recluse—even when I didn't feel like being social. At the same time, I said no when I needed to without feeling guilty. I tried to be honest with people about how I was feeling.

If you sense that the people around you are uncomfortable with your cancer, give them this book and tell them to read chapter 10, "What Can Family and Friends Do?" If your family still has difficulty accepting your diagnosis and offering support, seek out other friends or people in support groups who can be helpful. I even prayed specifically for God to bring people into my life who would be a source of strength to me. There are also doctors, counselors, and social workers today who specialize in helping a cancer patient cope.

It is normal to feel powerless in the face of cancer's threat. But while cancer will definitely change your life, it does not have to control it. You can fight back.

10
What Can Family and Friends Do?

It is easy to feel helpless and uncomfortable when someone you know and love has cancer. And many people respond by turning away because they just don't know what will help and what will only add to the hurt. While turning away may be the easy way out for you as a friend or family member, it is a terrible thing to do to a cancer patient. Following are some simple, specific ways you can offer support that really do make a difference:

Pray. And let the person know over and over that you are praying. Many people say a prayer when they first hear the news, or during the first surgery; but cancer is often a long drawn-out battle—a marathon rather than a sprint. Most of the time it requires not so much strength as endurance. Assure your friend faithfully of your continued prayers.

Give hugs freely and generously. There is nothing like a human touch to assure people that they are still alive and loved. Besides that, it may be easier for you if you can express your support without words.

Be optimistic. A cancer patient already feels weak and scared enough without being reminded of the odds or the side effects. Here are a few things I heard as a cancer patient that I really did not need to hear:

"Some make it; some don't."
"You're going to be a very sick girl."
"Oh, you'll probably lose your hair."
"Just think, you may be translated to glory soon."

Of course, all of the above observations were true. But at a time when I was struggling to *accept* my situation without *resigning* myself to it, they did more to harm my spirit than to help. Be honest and realistic with your cancer-patient friend without being totally negative. If you know any success stories, any friends who have *defeated* cancer, tell *those* to your friend. If you've experienced any miracles or other evidence of the power of prayer, share that. Remind yourself before you talk to your friend that cancer is not a death sentence. If you cannot make yourself believe this, just keep your opinion to yourself.

Also, avoid making comments about how your friend looks, unless you can honestly tell her she looks well. Cancer patients know when they look bad, so insincere compliments are not a comfort. Here is another list of things I did not need to hear about my appearance:

"Oh, you've lost so much weight. Are you feeling okay?"
"Your face is so puffy."
"Wow, you look tired."

A rule of etiquette that I read in a women's magazine applies to cancer patients as well as to everyone else: Bring to your friend's attention only those things she can do something about (like "Your slip is showing," not "Your hair's really getting thin").

Ask your friend if she wants to talk about it. Some people do; others don't. For many people, this is a time when they are feeling powerless anyway, so to have others intrude on their emotions and their privacy is an added difficulty. Others are simply waiting for someone to bridge the isolation they feel. Be sensitive to how your particular friend wants to handle communication.

What Can Family and Friends Do?

Don't introduce your friend to other people as "the cancer patient," as in, "Oh, this is Bea Hoek—she's the one I was telling you about who has cancer." Whether or not I have cancer, I want to be known for the person I am, not for the disease I happen to have.

If your friend is receptive, supply some good, Christian reading material or "how-to-cope-with-cancer" type books, or even accurate medical updates. But read the book yourself first to make sure it is positive and helpful, rather than discouraging. Also, be sensitive to your friend's level of energy. She may be too weak to read but would feel obligated to read what someone has given her. And be careful not to give your friend the impression that you have found a simple and definitive answer to her problem.

Don't be afraid to visit, but keep your visits short. Sometimes it exhausts a patient to carry on a conversation for more than twenty or thirty minutes. Ask your friend if she is getting tired. Hopefully, she will be honest enough to tell you that she's ready for a rest.

Although there were people I had to forgive for their insensitivity, I found that my network of friends and family played an important role in my recovery. Please do not be afraid of a friend's cancer. Have the courage to give your love and support. It may mean the difference between life and death.

11
Depression

The word *depression* is too small, too trite to convey the emotional darkness I as a cancer patient went through. In facing cancer I had to come to terms with the person I had been. I assessed the values I had spent my life forming and upholding. I was forced to try to imagine what death would be like—not just the actual physical *death* itself, but also the idea of not taking part in *life* anymore. For me this emotional side of cancer included vast loneliness, recurring hopelessness, and a lot of grief.

And dealing with all the humiliation and pain that are part of the illness as well as the cures, involves a lot of difficult emotions, too. I remember that during my chemo treatments it was always difficult for the nurse to get a vein, and more than once I found myself in tears of frustration. Sometimes, because of someone's incompetency, the needle would penetrate the tissue, and I could feel the chemicals burning.

I also remember visiting a local hair styling academy to be measured for a wig. I knew I more than likely would lose my hair, and I wanted to be prepared. Still, it was hard for me to face the idea of being bald, what I considered the ultimate insult. What is it about the sight of your own naked head that makes you feel vulnerable and transparent? I prayed that God would let me keep my hair.

But a cancer patient's battle with depression involves more than just emotions. There were chemical things at work in my body that affected my psychological well-being. The physical and emotional work closely together and are interdependent.

I tried hard to keep a positive attitude. I was having a hard time accepting the cancer's effects on my physical self; I did not want to concede the emotional battle as well. But the challenge was immense and frustrating, and I know I failed many times.

Add to that equation the chemicals I was taking orally and by injection. While they were vital to winning the physical battle, the drugs sometimes worked against me in the emotional battle. One of the drugs I was on was prednisone, a stimulant used to kill the cancer cells, prevent nausea, and reduce hair loss. My prescription called for 60mg each day for the five days during my chemo cycle. During those five days I was often very "up" and excited; in fact, the stimulant made it difficult for me to sleep more than five hours a night.

Then, at the end of the cycle, I came off all medication so that my blood count would return to normal. Having grown accustomed to the stimulating effects of the prednisone, being denied it so suddenly was like having a chair taken out from under my emotions. My mood darkened, my spirits plummeted. I felt devastated and alone.

Satan likes to attack us when we are weak and vulnerable, and he waged his cruel war with me every time I was mired in depression. He tempted me with self-pity and despair. He blinded me to God's promises and my family's faithfulness. He frustrated me with my own attempts to conquer my depression.

But God held me fast. As he always does.

I learned to plan something special with my friends for the day I was required to withdraw from the medication. I tried to fill the hours with activity and fun and people to ward off the emotional emptiness I knew was waiting for me. If I could depend on friends to get me through the two or three "empty" days, the struggle wasn't so draining.

Psalm 40

> I waited patiently for the Lord
> he turned to me and heard my cry.
> He lifted me out of the slimy pit,

Depression

out of the mud and mire;
he set my feet on a rock
and gave me a firm place to stand.
He put a new song in my mouth,
a hymn of praise to our God.
Many will see and fear
and put their trust in the LORD.

Blessed is the man
who makes the LORD his trust,
who does not look to the proud,
to those who turn aside to false gods.
Many, O LORD my God,
are the wonders you have done.
The things you planned for us
no one can recount to you;
were I to speak and tell of them,
they would be too many to declare.

Do not withhold your mercy from me,
O LORD;
may your love and your truth always protect me.
For troubles without number surround me;
my sins have overtaken me, and I cannot see.
They are more than the hairs of my head,
and my heart fails within me.

Be pleased, O LORD, to save me;
O LORD, come quickly to help me.

Yet I am poor and needy;
may the LORD think of me.
You are my help and my deliverer;
O my God, do not delay.

—verses 1–5, 11–13, 17

I also learned to hold my Father's hand through those empty days, knowing that only he could keep me from falling over the edge of the cliff I balanced on. I read and reread the promises I had marked in my Bible—promises of protection and redemption and returning joy.

In Psalm 40 David writes, "He lifted me out of the slimy pit, out of the mud and mire." I clung to that psalm during my periods of depression, desperately trusting God to lift me out of my own muddy pit.

Each time I suffered the pit of depression, each cycle I went through, with God's help I came out stronger. I learned things that I could take with me into the next cycle, and while I dreaded the darkness I knew I would face each time, I also came to know that the darkness would pass.

In a recent Chicago November we went through twenty-six consecutive days without sunshine. The skies were gray, and the rain was cold, but I hardly even noticed. Having known and conquered real darkness, a few cloudy days could have no effect on my spirits—not even twenty-six in a row!

"Lord, thank you for life—even in the dark, sunless days. Keep your Son shining in and through me. Amen."

12
Brought Low

Christmas 1983 was fast approaching. I had determined that this would be the best Christmas ever for my family. Even though I did not verbalize it, I wondered if it would be my last. Later, I found that others—my family and friends—wondered, too.

I was able to do some of my own Christmas shopping, though the trips were short because of my limited endurance. I remember trying to concentrate on details I had always known: What size does Jayne wear? What color did Jackie want? Was it a *black* leather belt Jon needed? It was difficult to think of anything but cancer for longer than ten minutes, and I was literally walking around in an annoying daze. In fact, the joyousness of the Christmas season actually seemed to lower my spirits rather than raise them. I heard people laughing and joking, and I morbidly thought, "I wish I had something to joke about."

Some of the family pictures I have of that Christmas dinner are rather grim reminders of that low time in my life. My face was swollen and puffy from the prednisone, and it was difficult for me to force a smile.

Still, I was determined to attend church as often as I could. In church I felt very close to God, and I was renewed by the support of fellow Christians. There were times when weakness forced me to remain seated during the singing, but the music strengthened my spirit. And never before had I been so thirsty for each word of each sermon. It seemed every pastor had a special message for me.

I went to church in the evening on Christmas day, although I could feel that my chemo treatment and general fatigue were beginning to affect me. During the service, nausea began to set in, and I got up to leave the sanctuary. My husband followed close behind me, which was fortunate because I didn't make it very far. I passed the organ in front of the church, but did not get to the swinging door just beyond before I fainted. When I recovered, I was lying on the floor in the hallway.

Paramedics were summoned, and their flashing lights and sirens seemed all the more urgent in the stillness of the church. Meanwhile, the pastor stopped his sermon and began to pray with the congregation.

At the hospital my embarrassment at fainting was combined with frustration. My worn-out veins were making it difficult for the nurses to start an IV. After three or four attempts, it was finally in place.

That night I wanted to pray, but I couldn't. God seemed far away, and I was too tired, too embarrassed, and too frustrated. I didn't know what to say or how to say it. There just were no words to sort out my feelings. I was physically, emotionally, and spiritually drained.

Out of the Depths I Cry

I wait for God, I trust his holy word;
　　he hears my sighs.
My soul still waits and looks unto the Lord;
　　my prayers arise.
I look for him to drive away my night—
　　yes, more than those who watch for morning light.

Hope in the Lord: unfailing is his love;
　　in him confide.
Mercy and full redemption from above
　　he does provide.
From sin and evil, mighty though they seem,
　　his arm almighty will his saints redeem.
　　　　　　　　　　—hymn based on Psalm 130
　　　　　　　　　　author unknown

That was a very low time in my life, but God did not leave me there. When I was too weak and overcome to even voice my feelings to him, he reminded me that his Holy Spirit intercedes for me "with groans that words cannot express." He also made me aware that my Christian family was lifting me up in prayer.

61

13
Scenes from the Radiation Waiting Room

I had been having chemo-therapy for a number of weeks and was scheduled to begin radiation treatments in January at Northwestern Hospital in Chicago. While I understood that the radiation was intended to make sure all the cancer was eradicated, I wondered how my body and mind would handle both treatments simultaneously. My oncologist regularly monitored my blood counts and adjusted my chemo doses based on what he found.

Before the radiation treatments could begin I had to be measured and prepared. It was a long, cold wait, on a hard table, with nothing but the ceiling tiles to look at. My whole upper left side was measured and marked with colored markers. Accuracy was important, so that the site where the tumor had been could be targeted for the most effective doses. Although the tumor was now gone, it was too early to know whether or not the cancer itself was. We could only complete all the treatments and then hope the final tests would show they had been effective.

A huge "linear accelerator machine"—known as a very specific, powerful, and effective machine—would administer the doses. Adjusting the machine and placing the protective lead wedges in just the right positions on my chest and throat took close to twenty minutes. I was scheduled for a regimen of twenty-eight days, taking breaks on Saturdays and Sundays.

A TV monitor in the technicians' station focused on me, so that the technicians could watch me at all times, even after they left the room to protect themselves from the radiation. At age forty-two I had become a television star—although this was not how I had pictured the life of a celebrity!

Alone in that cold, tiled room I felt far removed from the support of my friends and family. I felt alone with the cancer and shadowed by it. The powerful whine of the linear accelerator made me feel small.

Each of the twenty-eight treatments lasted only a minute or so, but I filled that minute with prayer. On the days when I was not asking for my own healing, I prayed for the fellow patients I had spent time with in the waiting room.

There was Betty, who also had breast cancer. She came for treatments on her lunch hours. She had become a widow only the year before, and knowing how much support I got from my husband, I felt her loss. Betty was a Christian, and she taught me a lot about dependence on God. "I don't even get out of bed in the morning without first talking to God," she told me. "It's the only way I can get through this." I found a lot of comfort in the spiritual bond that Betty and I formed.

A young mother came with her child of about eighteen months. The child was fussing and crying, obviously dreading what was ahead. His mother looked drained. It must have hurt her to know she would have to leave her son alone, restrained in the treatment room, without even being able to help him understand why. I'm sure she would rather have taken the treatment herself than put her baby through it.

Most everyone sat in silence, and most everyone was there alone—some by choice, and some by circumstance. I was able to have a different friend accompany me each day to ease the tension of waiting and to help pass the time. Other patients sometimes remarked how nice it was that my friends were so supportive.

I will never forget the young woman in the wheelchair. She suffered from lung cancer but was still addicted to cigarettes, so she passed her time coughing and smoking simultaneously. She was rather pretty, in spite of her illness, and she yearned for conversation. One day she asked me, "You come here in such good spirits—how do you manage that?" I told her that God was the source of my strength, courage, and perseverance, and that I talked to him continually. I offered to bring her some booklets she might find comforting. She seemed receptive. So I carefully prepared some materials which would speak to her present suffering as well as point the way to heaven.

The next day, for some reason, our treatments were not scheduled at the same time, so I didn't see her. The technicians told me she had been there already and had asked them to take the material I had for her and put it in her medical folder so she would get it the next day. I didn't see her after that, but I kept praying for her. When I came for a check-up a few months later, I asked about her. They told me she had died. Even though I could have expected that, I was stunned and sobered. I don't know if she found the comfort she needed, or if she accepted salvation before she faced the Lord.

That experience, combined with the whole awareness of mortality that cancer brings, really helped me put things in perspective. None of us know how long we will be here. None of us know whom we will meet, or exactly how God will use us. But if we are open to his preparation and leading, we just might be his instrument of choice for reaching someone who doesn't know him.

"Lord, please use me while I have the breath."

14
The Problem with Support Groups

$\mathcal{B}$*ecause cancer* is such a widespread problem today, many resources are out there to meet the needs of cancer patients. During my struggle I joined a number of different support groups. Some of them were unique and interesting, and many of them were very helpful, but I still felt a void—because all of the groups I tried lacked the spiritual dimension I desperately desired at the time. Since those early days I have found Christian groups which provide me with the spiritual strength I need, but back then I often felt very alone.

The Y-ME support group met in northwest Indiana, about forty-five minutes from my home. The meetings were informative and encouraging, and the interaction was healthy. Y-ME's goals were to promote discussion and communication among cancer patients, helping them to face their options honestly and knowledgeably. The woman who served as group leader at that time felt that silence feeds the fears we all face and that open communication helps dispel those fears.

Y-ME often hosted doctors, psychologists, nutritionists, and other health professionals, who shared with us their expertise and experience. I took a lot of notes and gained a deeper understanding of my situation. I also passed on this information to others.

It was at Y-ME that I met a woman named Sharon, through whom I got involved with another support group. Sharon was the director of a wellness clinic and had studied with a well-known oncologist, Dr. Carl Simonton, author of the book *Getting Well Again*. I found the group at the wellness clinic to be very caring and supportive, and the variety of lectures, seminars, and workshops offered was very helpful. I learned how to reduce stress, how to avoid being a "victim," how to change destructive thought patterns, etc. I also learned how to open up to others, sharing my own fears and trying to comfort them in theirs.

But I was frustrated because in this group I could not share the most important resource I had—my relationship with God. While most of the group members were interested in my faith, the leaders exclusively emphasized "the power within." (In fact, I was once told not to talk about God.) Their doctrine was that we can heal ourselves through positive thinking, visualization, or mental exercises. While I certainly believe that I have a power within myself which goes beyond science and medicine, I also *know* that that power comes *from God*, and it is only mine when I admit my own powerlessness. It's an odd paradox, I know, one which the apostle Paul expressed in 2 Corinthians 12: "But [God] said to me, 'My grace is sufficient for you, for my power is made perfect in weakness.' . . . For when I am weak, then I am strong" (vv. 9–10).

I was allowed to mention God in the group, and the others there knew that I consider him the source of my strength, but I was not allowed to elaborate like I wanted to. When someone in the group would share her feelings of isolation, I wanted to tell her that God never leaves us or forsakes us. When someone would describe frustration with people's inability to understand pain, I wanted to let that person know that my Savior suffered everything hell could throw at him, so he understands my cries as no one else can. When people would discuss their fears of death and dying, I wanted to share with them my hope and confidence in a future that goes beyond death, my complete assurance of the ultimate victory. But these things I was not allowed to share.

Scripture Guide

When you:

Are afraid	Deuteronomy 33:27 Isaiah 41:10 Romans 8:38–39
Are lonely	Deuteronomy 31:8
Are weary	Matthew 11:28
Are anxious	Philippians 4:6–7 1 Peter 5:7
Are depressed	Psalm 116
Need comfort	2 Corinthians 1:3–4 Psalm 23 Psalm 116
Need hope	1 Corinthians 15:42–44 Revelation 21:1–5

I do not want to say that their humanistic foundation made the support groups I joined valueless, but I felt a real need for Christian support groups. Christian doctors and health professionals must share not only their medical expertise but also their faith. And cancer patients who are Christians must seek each other out. If you are attending a secular support group, fine. Take from the group whatever good you can find, but don't let the group shake your Christian foundation.

15
Setback

"*Lord, here I am* again." February 1984 I was back in Decatur Memorial Hospital, being prepared for my radiation implant surgery. I was in my fourth month of chemotherapy, and the chemo treatments would continue for another five months. I had also gone through several weeks of external radiation treatment. My doctors felt that it was time now to add the internal radiation to my regimen. This, we hoped, would effectively complete our attack. Dr. McGee would perform the operation.

He examined the breast area and my left side, which were afflicted with raw, oozing burns where the radiation rays had bounced off the lead wedges. He soon concluded that the burns were too severe to allow him to proceed with the surgery. Instead he prescribed treatment for second degree burns and admitted me to the hospital.

Okay, Lord. I'm not angry. If this is the price I have to pay to be cancer free, I will endure it.

Dr. Burke, who had handled my earlier lymph node surgery, visited me. As an excellent surgeon who took pride in his meticulous work, he expressed his disappointment with this setback. "I know you were promised cosmetic results, and this doesn't exactly meet that criterion," he said. The burns would leave a nasty scar. I assured the good doctor that at this point I was not interested in cosmetic results; getting rid of the cancer was my top priority. But I thanked him for his concern.

The radiation implant surgery could take place after my burns had healed. The wait turned out to be about two weeks. My few days in the hospital allowed me to practice my positive attitude. In spite of the potential grief over the upset in my healing schedule, I could focus on the good things that were happening. The hospital room was comfortable. The care was excellent. I would have some time alone with my husband. I would get some much-needed rest. The situation was not all bad. And I would still get the radiation implants; I just had to wait a little longer.

From Thursday to Saturday I remained in the hospital, getting the dressings on my burns changed three times a day. Home on Saturday evening, I was able to make it to church the next day, the layers of salve, gauze, and tape hidden beneath my Sunday best. I was uncomfortable, but it felt good to be with the family of God again. I knew they had been praying for me, and I realized that it was probably those prayers that had kept me from despair or impatience with this setback.

"Father, thank you for your body of believers. This is what church is all about."

16
Total Surrender

$\mathcal{T}$omorrow would be my last chemo treatment. It was July, and by this time I had gone through nine months of tests, treatments, pain, and uncertainty. In the morning I would finally make my last trip downtown to the University of Chicago Hospital. I would sit in the same stale waiting room only once more. Tomorrow would be my last chemo treatment.

But I had to get through today first. Before I could get my final injection tomorrow, I would have to get a final blood count at the local clinic today. The blood counts always determined whether or not I would tolerate the next cycle of chemo.

For some reason, this was a very difficult day for me. My spirit and body were in rebellion. I had had enough! I felt drained and depleted. The medical technician tried several times but could not get a single vial of blood from my veins. The lymph node surgery had left my left arm sluggish and vulnerable, so it could not be used. The veins of my right arm were spent. I just could not bring forth any more blood. *"Enough, Lord!"* I cried to myself, *"I don't want to be here. It's been nine long months, and I can't take any more."*

My friend Alida was the nursing supervisor at the clinic. I asked for her, and she comforted me and brought me some orange juice. She could see that it was useless to try any longer, so she suggested that I wait until the next day and have my blood drawn at the university.

I knew my mind and body were not cooperating because I had reached my limit of endurance. My soul "groaned within me." I shed tears of frustration, and it felt good to cry. It relieved the tension. Wearily I drove home to get some rest. Tomorrow would be another day. *"Please, Lord, help my mind and body to cooperate."*

The next day arrived. I had spent some time during the night repeating "Thou wilt keep him in perfect peace whose mind is stayed on thee." And I had prayed, *"Please give me perfect peace, Lord; I can't do this without you. You've been with me this far. Please don't leave me now."*

My husband drove me downtown. As I arrived at Medicine 3A, I told the receptionist that I needed a blood count because I hadn't been able to produce enough blood for one the day before. I asked, "Can you recommend someone who is good at getting blood from worn out veins?" She told me to ask for Bendi. My husband and I walked down the hall to the blood lab, and I asked for Bendi. As I walked into the little room I told him, "I hear you're good." He smiled, "I'll try my best."

Bendi punctured my vein on the first try, and blood flowed freely into the three little vials. I praised him profusely and celebrated my last regular count procedure. *"Thank you, Lord, for being with me."*

I fairly bounced back to the chemo waiting room, confident that this too would go well—and it did. The oncology staff congratulated me on my last scheduled chemo treatment. What a milestone! Now it would be a three-month wait until the bone scan that would tell whether or not the treatments had done their work.

During the wait I began to feel tense and nervous. It had been a long haul, and I was so tired. The thought of the upcoming bone scan filled me with mixed emotions. I wanted to know, I just *had* to know! But the possibility of bad news made me want to put off knowing.

My husband and I had tried to develop a habit of walking a mile each day. These walks were important for me. I depended heavily on Jim's support, and during these walks we talked with each other and escaped from the world. Jim could always put my feelings into perspective without trivializing or judging them. Besides that, his unshakable conviction that I would be healed gave me a lot of strength.

I did, however, doubt from time to time. I guess I believed that God *could* heal me; I just didn't know if he *would*.

And now, having completed nine months of painful, time-consuming, emotionally draining treatments, and being forced to wait yet another three months to find out if it had all been worth it, I felt overcome. I couldn't handle the anxiety anymore, the wondering, the hoping, the waiting, the not knowing. I couldn't handle the anguished prayers and the lessons in trust and expectations. I couldn't handle being on the brink of mortality, just hovering.

So that day during our walk I gave it all up. I surrendered, totally, to God. I can show you the exact spot on the sidewalk where I stood with my husband and prayed, *"Lord, if you want me, please take me. I can't live with this fear and anxiety anymore. If you want me here, please make that plain to me, too. I trust you and accept whatever you have in store for me."*

And that was when I found peace.

I had felt glimmerings of that peace before—a sense of God's presence in the loneliness of the radiation room, an answer to a prayer for patience, the comfort and encouragement from people around me. But all of those glimpses were only fragments of the peace that was mine when I surrendered all of my hopes and fears and struggles to God. Now his peace filled my heart, calmed my mind, relaxed my body, and healed my soul. His peace was all-consuming and solidly powerful.

When Peace Like a River

When peace like a river attendeth my way,
when sorrows like sea billows roll;
whatever my lot, thou hast taught me to say,
"It is well, it is well with my soul."
—Horatio G. Spafford

That's the irony, I guess. I could only win the battle when I stopped fighting. Many cancer support groups and books and psychologists told me that the power to live, to defeat cancer, comes from within myself. But I know that's not completely true. The power that defeated my cancer came from God, and I was healed only when I admitted my own powerlessness.

Of course, surrendering to God does not mean throwing in the towel. Surrendering to God means opening oneself to his power, accepting the gift of his strength. There is a difference between giving in to God and giving in to the cancer, though the dividing line is very fine. I've had a hard time defining this difference, and perhaps the way I alternate—even today—between feelings of peace and feelings of anxiety, is evidence of that. Discovering God's will, and learning to trust it, is a lifelong exercise for every Christian. Throughout my battle with cancer, again and again, I had to bring myself back to an attitude that said, *"Lord, I want you to heal me. But if you choose not to, help me to believe that that's okay, too."*

Another part of the Christian struggle is to know *when* or *how* or *how often* to ask God for what we want. Too often we come *timidly* before the throne of grace because we are afraid that our petition will not fall within God's plan for us. As the old prayer says, "Lord, grant me the serenity to accept the things I cannot change, the courage to change the things I can, and the wisdom to know the difference."

I like that prayer, but maybe to reflect an attitude of total surrender it should say instead, "Lord, grant me the serenity to accept the things you will not change, the courage to trust you to change the rest to work out for my good, and the wisdom to know the difference."

The most important lesson I have learned throughout the past ten years is the lesson that Paul teaches in his second letter to the Corinthians: "But [God] said to me, 'My grace is sufficient for you, for my power is made perfect in weakness.' Therefore I will boast all the more gladly about my weaknesses, so that Christ's power may rest on me. That is why, for Christ's sake, I delight in weaknesses, in insults, in hardships, in persecutions, in difficulties. For when I am weak, then I am strong" (2 Cor. 12:9–10).

Peter says it well, too, "Humble yourselves, therefore, under God's mighty hand, that he may lift you up in due time" (1 Peter 5:6).

Total Surrender

It would be nice if total surrender were a one-time event, a milestone indicating completion or accomplishment. But of course it is not. It is a process. That day in July was only the beginning, and that place on the sidewalk marked only the first step. For the rest of my life now I have to drag myself back—daily, sometimes *hourly*—to the altar of sacrifice and surrender my life to God again.

17
God's Answer

My journal entry for the day before my bone scan says simply, "Very uptight." I thought about this the following morning as, filled with radioactive dye and numerous glasses of liquid, I lay quietly on the steel table at the hospital. I compared that entry with my feelings three months ago when I had found peace by totally surrendering myself to God. It seemed so long ago. Was that peace still there? I had to keep reminding myself that it was, as long as I continued to put my trust in God. *"He has heard your prayers, Bea,"* I said to myself, *"and you can trust him for the perfect answer."*

This was perhaps the hardest sacrifice I had to make. How could I surrender my desire to *live*, to be healthy again? I wanted so desperately for God to answer my prayers the way *I* wanted. I did not want to hear him if his plan was different from mine. I didn't want to accept a negative report. I pictured myself putting my hands over my ears and squeezing my eyes shut, afraid of hearing something I didn't want to hear.

The bone scan seemed to last forever, though in reality it took only an hour. That was just the time I needed to drag myself to the altar of sacrifice again. When the test was over, I was feeling God's peace renewed in my spirit.

Now I had to wait one more day for God's answer to my three months of prayer. The test results would be in tomorrow, and Jim and I would meet with Dr. Vogelzang to find out if the cancer had been eradicated.

We prayed together the next morning before driving down to the hospital. We asked for healing, and for peace, but most of all for the faith to totally surrender again. It is so hard to let go and let God! It just goes against every natural instinct, even though I *know* things will only turn out better if I do.

The time Jim and I spent in the waiting room seemed in one sense to drag, and yet, in another sense, I couldn't believe it when my name was called so quickly. This was it—the moment of revelation, the unveiling of the answer to my prayers. It almost didn't seem real.

We entered Dr. Vogelzang's small office and accepted the two available chairs. Hardly daring to breathe, I watched him open my file, adjust his glasses, and glance over the materials inside. He frowned in mock concentration, then looked at me and smiled. "The scan came back normal," he reported. "I am giving you a clean bill of health."

"Praise the Lord!" was all I could say, and I blinked back tears as the waves of relief swept over me. It was over—the battle was over. The cancer was gone!

That night, after calling relatives and friends with the good news, I faced the blank page of my daily journal. "Wednesday, October 31, 1984," I wrote. Then I sat back and thought for a while. What could I say? How could I capture this day on paper? Were there any words big enough or dramatic enough or beautiful enough to tell my story?

I smiled and sighed and wrote a simple *"Hallelujah."*

18
Living with Uncertainty

It is July 1992, eight years after my "Hallelujah" day. I have a tight feeling in my chest, and I don't want to jump to conclusions or be overly anxious, but I'm nervous. I've been having a lot of pain in my left arm and shoulder, and I'm not sure what that means. It seemed for so long that my life was back to normal—and now this.

I don't know if this is God's way of teaching me complete dependence, or of reminding me not to start taking things for granted again, or what—do I really need another lesson?

It seems the cancer experience is never over. The sickness itself can drag on for years. The various cures and treatments last for months at a time. And then, even when you're cured, there is always the possibility of recurrence.

Twice a year I return to the University of Chicago medical center for a bone scan. The two or three weeks prior to the scan are usually filled with the same kind of nervousness and tension that I used to feel in high school the day before a big test. My mind races with questions and doubts: Have I been eating right? Should I be exercising more? Is that a normal bruise, or does it mean something? The shadow of uncertainty does not lift until nearly a week after the test, when I finally get the results. If the scan is clear, I can breathe a sigh of thanks and go on with my "normal" life again.

But this time the shadow did not lift right away. When I called for the results of my scan, I was told that a spot had shown up on my sternum. Stunned and battling a sick feeling in my stomach, I made an appointment with Dr. Vogelzang.

He greeted me with a grim seriousness that was unusual for him. The spot was not necessarily cancer, but he did not want to take any chances. He called for more tests and consultations with a team of doctors and specialists. He also prescribed a new medication called tamoxifen. Besides being afraid, I was bitterly disappointed. I had been praying for a clean bill of health.

Both of the follow-up bone scans I underwent during the next six months continued to show the spot on my sternum. It was still there, but it had not grown any larger. I thanked God for that.

Then in December I went back for a third bone scan, prepared for the same results. But this time the tests came back clear.

"Do you think the tamoxifen is responsible?" I asked Dr. Vogelzang incredulously at his office.

"It could be," he answered. "But you and I both know what else it could be. Our powerful God can erase any spot, or heal any disease, or ease any uncertainty." I nearly cried with joy and relief.

This is the kind of uncertainty I live with every day now. It is a frustrating test of my willingness to totally surrender. Even when I think I'm cured, the threat of recurrence is there. My semiannual bone scan reminds me that, in a sense, I never leave the valley of the shadow of death. My life now is never my own; I can never regain the feeling of control that I had before I got cancer.

Maybe that's good. None of us really control our own lives, though we like to think we do. And while it's frustrating for me to have to be continually reminded of my mortality, it's an important lesson to learn. God is in control. My very existence is a gift of his will. I am *nothing* apart from him. He measures out each breath I take. He carefully calculates each beat of my heart. Without his hand constantly around me, I would simply collapse.

It took cancer to make me aware of that. Constantly aware of it.

The Difference

My footsteps echo off the stone and cold
and, magnified in contrast with the still,
re-shatter my already broken will.
I sit,
        and feel the hallowed hollow fill
and slowly heal my stubborn, hollow soul.

A seed must die before it can be born.
The old must pass before the new can come.
And as I tremble—
        crumbled, humbled, numb—
a shaft of sunrise speaks the broken morn.

—M. J.

As I've said before, the hardest thing to live with is the waiting. But each time a new uncertainty arises— whether it's an abnormality that shows up on a scan, or just an odd feeling that something may not be right—I learn again to "wait patiently for the Lord."

"Lord, teach me gentleness in the face of disappointment. And help me to profit by the suffering that comes my way. Amen."

19
Easter

I love *Easter.* I suppose a lot of people do. Most people know the Easter story—they have heard about it in church, told it to their kids, even seen it on TV. But still, if it's only a story to you, then you're missing the point.

The significance of Christ's death is this: He died so we don't have to.

Jesus' resurrection is one of the most important things Christians believe. Our faith is worthless unless we know that Jesus rose from the dead. *His* victory over death allows *our* victory. There is no life outside of the life he won for us.

Jesus conquered death. And he empowers us with the same strength. We are no longer threatened by death because we can conquer it, too. Jesus' victory means not only a powerful life for us here on earth, but also an unending, perfect life in heaven.

It's easy to forget about the meaning of Easter when we are caught up in the "dailyness" of everyday life. And it's easy to forget the meaning of Easter when death and pain stare us in the face, trying to make us back down.

But Easter Sunday makes the power real again. I sat in church one Easter, surrounded by waves of glorious music and a circle of joyful saints. I sang the songs and prayed the hallelujahs. I listened to the story and knew again that it was meant for *me.*

We all need Easter. Whether we realize it or not, we all depend on what Christ did for us not only *on* the cross, but also *after* the cross.

I love Easter.

> He smiled at our amazement,
> and his eyes were laughing bright.
> He showed the jagged nail-scars, and we trembled at the
>   sight.
> But suddenly my grief and guilt were more than I could
>   stand;
> I turned away to fight the tears—
>   but he held out his hand.
>
> The hand that healed the leper now reached out to
>   make *me* whole;
> the scars that marked his body matched the wounds
>   upon my soul.
>
> Death's power once had bound him, and bound *us* in
>   misery,
> but in his resurrection Jesus resurrected me.
>   —M. J., in *Easter*

20
Thank You, Lord

It's a shame that we fully appreciate the things we have and the people we love only when we are afraid of losing it all. It's so easy to take life for granted—until we are faced with death.

My embarrassment at my former apathy does not keep me from expressing my thanks now. I want to list some of the things I have learned to appreciate again, and maybe my list will remind you of some of the good things in your own life.

Thank you, Lord, for my church. It is good to have a place to go where people are not afraid to show they love me, where friends do their best to understand me, where I can be involved in things that are both fun and meaningful. Thank you for my time in the choir—for good Christian fellowship, and for beautiful words and music.

Thank you, Lord, for special friends who are willing to share my burdens, who do not feel self-conscious about sharing their own. Thank you for people I can trust with a secret.

Facing the Unknown

Are you afraid of the future?
Do you wonder what life holds for you?
There is, it seems, a lot to worry about.

Will I be completely abandoned?
Will I beat this thing?
How bad will my situation get before I die?
And what will happen after I die?

Facing the unknown is always disturbing—
and often terrifying.
But if your heart belongs to God,
you can see beyond your situation today.
You can know
for sure
what your future holds.

Trust Jesus.
He died and went through hell
to heal all our diseases
and bring us back to life.

He took the sting out of death
and the fear out of the future.

Let him fill you with his peace
   and comfort you with his promises.

Besides giving you confidence in your eternal destiny,
trusting your
tomorrows
to him
can give you the strength you need
to face anything
today.

—M. J., in *Never Too Late*

Thank you, Lord, for the everyday celebrations of life. Thank you that birthdays and weddings and family reunions go on.

Thank you for my job. As a substitute teacher, I feel the importance of my work, and I enjoy shaping the lives you put in my care. Thank you for my co-workers, people who are good at what they do and know how important it is. Thank you for a wise and responsible administration. Thank you most of all for children. Their honesty and eagerness and undisguised joy are refreshing.

Thank you, Lord, for Jim. Thank you for the concerts and operas we enjoy together. Thank you for how comfortable we feel with each other. Thank you for his quiet strength and firm faith in you. Every day we become closer friends.

Thank you for my children—for the joy they have brought me and the support they have been to me. Thank you for allowing me to enjoy the milestones of their lives. Thank you, too, for the special mates you have blessed them with.

Years ago I prayed that you would spare me, Lord, so that I could enjoy my grandchildren. Thank you for your answer to that prayer. Lord, I love my grandchildren. Thank you for the fun we have together, for the energy you give me to keep up with them! Thank you for the love they have for you already. Lord, my heart overflows with your promises and your goodness. Thank you for my grandchildren.

Thank you, too, for my parents who love you, and who still share that love with me. They have always been available to me when I need them, and they are prayer warriors who help me in my spiritual battle.

Thank you, Lord, for your peace. I really don't have to be afraid. Thank you for having the patience to teach me, over and over, that I can trust you. Lord, I believe. Help me overcome my unbelief.

Lord, thank you for life. For this life here on earth, yes, but even more for the promise of life in heaven that will never end. You are my rock, my hope, my salvation, the only thing worth having. Lord, I love you.

Appendix

Resources Cancer Patients May Find Helpful

Literature

Becton, Randy. *Everyday Strength: A Cancer Patient's Guide to Spiritual Survival*. Grand Rapids: Baker, 1989.

Benjamin, Harold H. *From Victim to Victor*. New York: Dell, 1987.

Bloch, Annette and Richard. *Fighting Cancer*. Kansas City, Missouri: Cancer Connection, Inc., 1985.

Collins, Gary. *Spotlight on Stress*. Santa Ana, California: Vision House, 1983.

Cousins, Norman. *Anatomy of an Illness*. New York: Bantam, 1983.

Diamond, Harvey and Marilyn. *Fit for Life*. New York: Warner Books, 1987.

Hoeksema, Herman. *Meditations: God Is Our Refuge and Strength*. Grand Rapids, 1946. (Copies obtained by writing South Holland Protestant Reformed Church, 16511 South Park Avenue, South Holland, Illinois 60473.)

Jaffe, Dennis. *Healing from Within*. New York: Simon and Schuster, 1986.

Jongsma, Melanie. *Hope in the Face of Death*. South Holland, Illinois: The Bible League, 1991.

———. *Stress: Letting Go and Letting God*. South Holland, Illinois: The Bible League, 1993.

———. *Talking with God*. South Holland, Illinois: The Bible League, 1992.

Larson, Bruce. *There's a Lot More to Health Than Not Being Sick*. Waco, Texas: Word Books, 1984.

Little, Bill L. *Help Yourself Heal: Eight Steps to Health and Wholeness*. Minneapolis: CompCare Publishers, 1990.

Meier, Paul D. *Meditating for Success*. Grand Rapids, Michigan: Baker Book House, 1978.

Minirth, Frank B., and Paul D. Meier. *Happiness Is a Choice: a Manual on the Symptoms, Causes, and Cures of Depression*. Grand Rapids, Michigan: Baker Book House, 1978.

Reisser, Paul. *Energy Drainers, Energy Gainers*. Grand Rapids, Michigan: Zondervan, 1990.

Roels, Edwin D. *Someone Cares: Scripture Truths for Those Who Are Ill*. South Holland, Illinois: The Bible League, 1982.

Salaman, Maureen. *Nutrition: The Cancer Answer*. Menlo Park, California: Statford Publishing, 1989.

Siegel, Bernie S. *Love, Medicine, and Miracles*. New York: Harper & Row, 1990.

Simonton, O. Carl, and Stephanie Simonton. *Getting Well Again*. Los Angeles: Bantam Books, 1982.

U.S. Department of Health and Human Services. *Chemotherapy and You: a Guide to Self-Help During Treatment*. National Institute of Health Publications: National Cancer Institute, 1990.

Appendix

U.S. Department of Health and Human Services. *Taking Time.* National Institute of Health Publications, 1990.

Vanderwell, Howard D. *Proven Promises.* Hudsonville, Michigan, 1990.

Support Groups and Hotlines

The American Cancer Society
1-800-ACS-2345
777 Third Avenue
New York, NY 10017
   (local units are listed in your telephone
   directory)

The National Cancer Institute
1-800-4-CANCER

Y-ME
1-800-221-2141